GYNECOLOGY

GYNECOLOGY

THREE MINIMALLY INVASIVE PROCEDURES YOU
NEED TO KNOW ABOUT FOR:

Permanent Birth Control,
Heavy Menstrual Periods,
Accidental Loss of Urine

PLUS:

Modern Hormone Therapy for the Post Menopausal Women

Dr. Maurice Leibman
MD, MSc, FACOG, FACS

Library of Congress Control Number: 2012902507
ISBN: Hardcover   978-1-4691-6537-0
                 Softcover   978-1-4691-6536-3
                 Ebook   978-1-4691-6538-7

This book was printed in the United States of America.

To order additional copies of this book, contact:
Xlibris Corporation
1-888-795-4274
www.Xlibris.com
Orders@Xlibris.com
104646

CONTENTS

Chapter One

Chapter Two

Chapter Three

Chapter Four

CHAPTER ONE

PERMANENT BIRTH CONTROL

Here are some facts that should grab your attention.

40% of pregnancies in the United States are unintended. This may come as a surprise to you, but for women over the age of 40—the rate is 51%. One third of pregnancies are in women who consider their families complete.

Permanent birth control is used in only 18% of women aged 15 to 44 years, who have completed their families, in the United States.

There are approximately one million procedures performed for perment birth control in the U.S. annually.

It is the third most common female surgery, following cesarian section and hysterectomy. The "tubal ligation" of the past has been surpassed by the **Essure** permanent birth control procedure, which is now the standard of care.

Laparoscopic tubal ligation is the most common performed procedure for sterilization, and even today is typically performed under general anesthesia in a hospital or outpatient facility. Although this is generally safe and effective, it carries some noteworthy risks related to the procedure itself and anesthesia, and the cost is significant in time and money. It is outdated and not considered to be on par with the more modern techniques that you will read about.

Permanent birth control has changed from being a costly major surgery in the hospital or surgicenter to a **minimally invasive office procedure** that takes approximately 10 minutes in the office, and has a recovery time of less than a day.

In November 2002, the FDA approved *Essure* for permanent birth control. **Essure is a nonincisional occlusion of the fallopian tubes that does not require general anesthesia, no cutting, no hormones and can be done in the office setting.** Advantages include decreased post procedural pain, decreased risk of adjacent organ/tissue damage, and more rapid recovery time.

The Essure procedure consists of inserting microcoils containing nickel, titanium, stainless steel, and polyethylene fibers into the Fallopian tubes. These microcoils use the body's natural healing response to block the Fallopian tubes, resulting in permanent birth control.

This simple procedure does not require incisions, contains no hormones, and women never have to worry about birth control again. There are over 300 publications in medical journals describing positive experience with the Essure procedure, so the safety and efficacy are well documented.

To date approximately 650,000 Essure procedures have been done in over 30 countries world wide, with a no pregnancy rate of 99.7% in the 10 year published data, when placed correctly. At this time the Essure procedure is the most effective, safest and least expensive form of female or male sterilization, as it surpasses even vasectomy, as a form of non reversible family planning

After three months, the Essure Confirmation Test is performed to confirm and document the satisfactory microinsert location as well as tubal occlusion in both tubes to satisfy the FDA requirement.

A study published in BJOG (British Journal of Obstetrics and Gynecology 2005) looked at **patient satisfaction** with Essure vs. the older (and regrettably still performed laparoscopic tubal ligation) and showed that at 90 days post-procedure, 100% of the women in the Essure group were "very satisfied" with their speed of recovery versus 80% in the laparoscopic sterilization group. The data from 2011 publications confirms this 2005 data.

What about the fluid used to distend the uterus during the procedure?

The uterine cavity is a potential space, which means it is not really an empty cavity at all ! The thick muscular walls of the uterus are in a collapsed state when the uterus is not pregnant, so a fluid is needed to distend the uterine cavity to visualize the inside. Normal saline is simply allowed to run in by gravity from an IV bag hung on a pole, and is not harmful in anyway to the body as it is a physiological solution. Almost all the fluid that is put into the uterus is recovered and discarded.

The insertion

The Essure micro-insert is a dynamically expanding 4-cm long microcoil that consists of a stainless steel inner coil, an expanding super-elastic outer coil, and polyethylene (Dacron) (PET) fibers.

The vagina is cleaned with Betadine (or Chlorhexidene if allergic to Betadine) and the hysteroscope introduced into the vagina. (vaginoscopy). The saline flow is turned on and the vagina fills with fluid and the cervix easily seen. The hysteroscope is then passed through the cervix with hydro-distention, into the uterine cavity and the opening of the tube on both sides confirmed. The Essure catheter is then passed through the hysteroscope and the microcoils placed one a time in the Fallopian tubes. Visual confirmation of the appropriate placement of the Essure microcoils is immediately seen on the monitor screen. Often during the procedure, our patients will be comfortable enough to watch their own insertion and deployment as it happens on the monitor ! This is similar to placing a heart stent and the technology is much the same. The PET fibers cause a benign inflammatory response along 3-4 cm of the inner tube, that results in the microcoil staying in place, causing a mechanical obstruction of the tubes and preventing pregnancy.

These PET coils were chosen as a result of their effectiveness in other clinical settings, such as arterial grafts in cardiac surgery, percutaneous catheters, and aneurysm coils as in brain surgery.

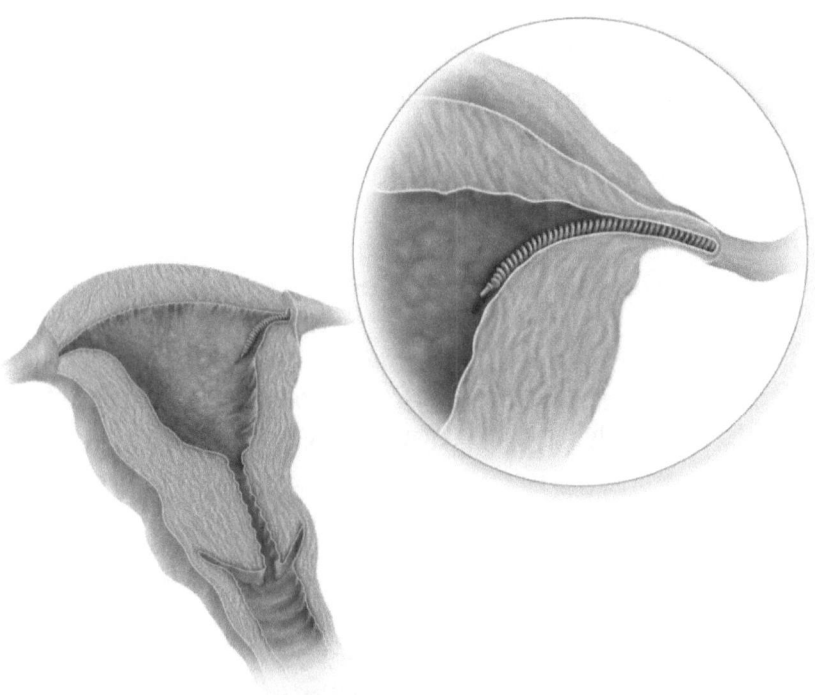

Essure microcoil in Fallopian tube

HOW DOES ESSURE WORK?

Soft, flexible inserts are placed into the Fallopian tubes as described above. No incision is needed because these tiny inserts are delivered through the vagina and cervix to the Fallopian tubes, much the same way as a heart stent is placed in a coronary artery.Over the next three months, a natural barrier forms around the inserts and prevents sperm from reaching the eggs. The ovaries will continue to release eggs, but the eggs will be absorbed back into the body, and not cause any harm.

Trailing Coils

The manufacturer recommends that 3-8 "trailing coils" be visible after the device is placed. These are the loops that are visible at the end of the device and can easily be seen and counted on the monitor screen on completion of the insertion. These trailing coils become covered in tissue (encapsulated) over time, and are not exposed in the uterine cavity. There can be as many as 18 trailing coils exposed in the uterine cavity, and it still be effective and safe. If there are 18 coils exposed it still means that more than half the coils are in the right place in the Fallopian tube and it will be effective.

The major strength of the Essure is the very high success rate—0% failure in clinical trials over 10 years, great patient satisfaction, low cost, and less than one day recovery time.

The Confirmation Test

After three months, it's time to get the Essure confirmation test to confirm the tubes are blocked and you don't have to worry about an unplanned pregnancy. A special type of x-ray with a dye is done (hysterosalpingogram) to ensure that the implants are in the right place and that the Fallopian tubes are completely blocked. Until that time, you must continue to use another form of birth control. This x-ray is read by a radiologist specially trained in this type of procedure and the result sent to your doctor.

Can I be put to sleep for the Essure?

Yes, you can! A board certified anesthesiologist comes to our office and can put you to sleep for the 10 minutes or so that the entire procedure takes. You will be carefully monitored during the anesthesia and will wake with a clear head. When you are awake and alert and comfortable, you must have someone drive you home. Once you get home, I recommend something to eat, some pain medication if necessary, then a nap! Once you wake from the nap, you should be able to do whatever you want.

What about allergy to Nickel?

Nickel allergy is the most common metal allergy and affects approximately 1 in 5,000 patients (1/5000). The most important risk factors for developing nickel sensitivity are female gender and younger age. Nickel is found in jewelry, eye glass frames, watch bands, belt buckles, snaps, and coins. The diagnosis of nickel allergies usually presents as a rash that looks like eczema or small raised red lesion that look like bumps.

For patients with a nickel sensitivity, alternative forms of birth control can be discussed, however Nickel allergy is not a contraindication to the insertion of Nickel and has recently been removed from the contraindication list by the manufacturer.

There is only one reported case of Nickel sensitivity as of February 2011. If Nickel hypersensitivity is confirmed after placement of the microcoils, removal is possible up to 6 weeks after the initial placement by simply inserting the hysteroscope, just as in the placement of the device, and pulling it out.

Expulsion and Perforation of the Micro devices

In the clinical trials for Essure, **a perforation rate** (microcoil going right through the tube) **of 1.8% occurred and an expulsion rate** (microcoils expelled from the tubes) **2.2% occurred.**

Nine women with expulsion of the Essure device in the clinical trials elected to undergo repeat procedures with subsequent success.

No additional surgery is needed to remove a device if it perforates through the tube into the abdominal cavity or into the muscle of the uterus. The device is so small it becomes encapsulated and does not harm or cause pain.

Seldom Offered Information

In a study of 645 women, overall placement success in both tubes at the first attempt was achieved in 95%, so there are times when for technical reasons it is just not possible to get both tubes blocked. **No procedure is always sucessful no matter who does it !** With the Essure there is never a 100% guarantee that it will work, but there is a very high probability that it will. ! Sometimes your anatomy is just not picture perfect and the openings to the fallopian tubes are difficult to find. The main reason for not being able to see and cannulate both tubes is when the tubes are located in an unusual position, for example, on the side of the uterus instead of the top of the uterus, or when you are born with a tilted uterus (retroverted) Also, difficulty in placing the micro-coils may result from tubal spasm that occurs in some people, or from blockage of the tubes from a prior tubal infection (pelvic inflammatory disease). We have started to use a muscle relaxant under the tongue if spasm occurs, and it seems to work. This is uncommon, but can happen.

Adverse events reported on the day of treatment procedure, include cramping, vaginal spotting, pelvic pain, nausea, back pain, headache. These occur in less than 2% of our patients.

Adverse events during the next 12 month

Menstrual cramping, headaches, back pain, heavy bleeding, vaginal spotting can occur. All the above are very uncommon and occurred in less than 2%. Sometimes these symptoms occur even if no surgery is performed!

What happens if the confirmation test at 3 months post procedure shows one or both tubes are still open?

The radiologist who performs and interprets the confirmation test will alert your physician if one or both tubes are not occluded. You and your doctor will then decide to repeat the Essure or go to the laparoscopic tubal ligation.

What other permanent birth control options are there?

At this time (2011) the only other FDA approved minimally invasive procedure for permanent birth control is the **Adiana**. It is similar to the Essure and results in a mechanical blockage of the fallopian tubes as well.

With the Adiana, a flexible instrument is passed through the cervix into the uterine cavity to deliver a tiny insert (size of a grain of sand) to a very specific location in the tube (cornu), and then a small amount of energy is delivered to the insert. The body's own tissue will grow in and around the tiny, soft inserts. After three months, just like the Essure procedure, a confirmation test (HSG) is performed to confirm that the tubes are blocked.

The problem with the Adiana procedure at this time is that it is less effective than the Essure. The engineering of this device may be flawed and it is more difficult for the physician to get skilled at doing it. No doubt it will be revised and improved in the future.

The official data rates contraceptive failures per 1000 women at year 3 as:

Essure: 1.6
Adiana: 16.0
Tubal Ligation: 9.9

Laparoscopic Tubal Ligation (BTL)

This old favorite is definitely now out of date. This procedure is what residents are taught during the early training phases of their careers to develop their laparoscopic skills.

There are a couple of occlusion devices used to block the tubes with the laparoscopic approach, such as cauterization, fallope rings, and spring clips.

While all three do the job, the failure rate is higher, cost higher and potential risk for injury higher and therefore not acceptable. Also, the additional cost of time, hospitalization or outpatient surgery center are considerable when compared to the minimally invasive procedures, like the Essure and Adiana.

The laparoscopic BTL has the additional risk of injury to the bladder, bowel, and major blood vessels in the abdomen when the instruments are inserted through the abdomen. The post-operative recovery is significantly more difficult and more painful too, up to a week in most cases.

At this time, the most favorable procedure for permanent birth control for minimal discomfort, efficiency, cost, and patient satisfaction is the Essure. As time passes, the Essure may be surpassed by something better and cheaper or perhaps just an updated version of the same technology making it simpler for the physician to insert and even less uncomfortable for the patient, but the principle of minimally invasive technique and technology is here to stay.

A report just released in February 2012 describes two patients who underwent a reversal of the ESSURE procedure. The first was a 37 year old who had the micrcoils inserted 5 years earlier, and the second was a 26 year old who had the procedure done one year earlier. Both had successful removal of the microcoils with subsequent pregnancies of normal term babies. I believe this is the first report of a successful pregnancy following removal of the microcoils.

While it is clearly emphasized in many places in this chapter that The ESSURE is a permanent birth control technique this is certainly interesting information.

Contraceptive Failures per 1000 Women at Year 3:

Essure: 1.6
Tubal Ligation: 9.9
Vasectomy   11.3
Adiana   16.0

To put contraception in a broader perspective, typical first year failure rate of commonly used contraception include

16% for the diaphragm, 15% for condoms, 8% for oral contraceptive pills, and 3% for the DepoProvera shot.

The Essure transcervical procedure is made and distributed by Conceptus Inc., San Carlos, CA, and was approved by the United States Food and Drug Administration in November 2002.

In Summary:

Can I trust the Essure procedure?

The Essure is 99.74% effective with zero pregnancies in ten years of clinical trials, making it the most effective method of permanent birth control available.

Is it painful?

Some women report discomfort or cramping as the microcoils are deployed into the tubes. Everyone has a different threshold for pain. Generally speaking, it is very well tolerated.

How long is the recovery?

Women are typically able to go home within 30 minutes of having the procedure, and the majority of women return to normal activities the next day. In fact, some of our patients have gone to their kids baseball or football game the same evening, a couple hours after the procedure.

Is it reversible?

No, the Essure procedure is not reversible, like the tubal ligation or vasectomy. Essure is permanent, so you should be sure your family is complete.

Will I still have a period?

Yes, you will still have a period, though some Essure users find that their period changes afterward, becoming slightly lighter or heavier. These changes may be the result of discontinuing birth control pills and returning to your natural cycle.

Is Essure covered by my insurance?

The Essure procedure is covered by most health insurance providers. If the Essure procedure is performed in a doctor's office, depending on your specific insurance plan, payment may be as low as a simple co-pay.

Is it safe?

The Essure procedure avoids the risks and discomfort of surgical procedures like tubal ligation and vasectomy. Additionally, the silicone-free inserts are made from materials that have been used successfully for many years in cardiac stents and other medical devices that are placed in the body.

References:

Obstetrics & Gynecology 2003; 102: 59-67

U.S. Food and Drug Administration. FDA talk paper. FDA approves new female sterilization device. November 4, 2002.

Trussell J. Contraceptive Efficacy. In: Hatcher RA, et al Contraceptive Technology, 19th Revised ed. New York (NY): Ardent Medium. 2007

CHAPTER TWO

HEAVY PERIODS

Heavy menstrual bleeding is a common gynecological condition that can seriously disrupt daily living. Not only will it affect adversely the quality of life for this "period" each month, but significant resources are used up with repeated visits to the gynecologist, refills on birth control pills or other medications to make the period acceptable. In more than 50% of cases, no pathology is found, so we call it "dysfunctional uterine bleeding," meaning we just don't know!

The first treatment usually recommended, is birth control pills or Lysteda (tranexamic acid), or NSAID's (nonsteroidal anti-inflammatory drugs) and when that fails **endometrial ablation** is indicated. [Obstetrics and Gynecology Vol. 117, No 1, Jan 2011]. There are however, many potential side effects from these medications, such as headaches, fatigue, loss of libido, vaginal spotting, nausea, breast tenderness, joint pain, muscle cramps, and easy bruising.

More than 1 in 5 women suffer from heavy periods and if you find you are scheduling your life around your period each month, you're not alone. In this new age of "**minimally invasive surgery**" we are now able to offer a choice for women that is simple, safe and extremely effective. You don't have to live with heavy periods or take medication every day or during your period, to alleviate the heavy bleeding. There is a simple, safe, and effective solution that takes about 90 seconds that is highly successful and has great patient satisfaction.

Consider the following:

Your family is complete
Your periods last 7 days or longer.
Your bleeding so heavy that you need to change your pad or tampon every 1 to 2 hours.
Cramping during your period requires medication or at least the desire for something to lesson the pain.
You often wear a tampon AND a pad for more protection. You pass clots.
You are tired during your period or anemic from repeated heavy flows.
Your bleeding affects your work, social, athletic, or sexual activities.
Your life would improve if you had less bleeding or no bleeding each month.
You are fed up with irregularity of perimenopausal bleeding.
Your periods associated with irritability and other PMS symptoms.

The facts

Clinical studies show that heavy bleeding and pain exist together in up to 93% of women with heavy bleeding (menorrhagia).

31% of women report missing school or work and 40% report social withdrawal and sexual avoidance due to pain.

Of the estimated 10 million women who suffer from heavy menstrual bleeding, only 2.5 million seek treatment each year. The reason for this is that many women "just put up with it," are "embarrassed" to discuss their periods, and they think their bleeding is normal because it has always been so heavy and they are afraid of treatment.

Heavy bleeding and cramping is common after a **tubal ligation** for permanent birth control (where the tubes are cauterized or banded and the blood supply to the ovaries and uterus is compromised).

Perimenopausal bleeding (women approaching the menopause) can be abnormal, frustrating, heavy, and irregular.

Women with **endometriosis** of the uterus, called adenomyosis, have especially painful menses often associated with heavy bleeding.

Approximately 22% of gynecological referrals are related to **menstrual disorders**.

In the United States alone, it is estimated that menorrhagia (or heavy menstrual bleeding) is responsible for about 1 billion dollars in direct costs and 12 billion dollars in indirect costs annually.

Additionally, approximately 30% of the 600,000 hysterectomies performed annually in the United States are for heavy menstrual bleeding.

Knowing that there is a simple, safe, and effective solution that takes about 90 seconds for the **Novasure** procedure and about 10 minutes with the **Thermachoice** procedure (both done in the office), may inspire you to consider this remarkable solution of endometrial ablation, and start the conversation with your doctor about what might be your choice for a conservative approach to your heavy bleeding.

Why something new? The need for a new way of treating heavy menstrual flow with and without cramps has always been obvious. Hormone treatment with birth control pills or NSAID (nonsteroidal anti-inflammatory drugs) has been the mainstay forever, and if that did not work, then hysterectomy. The hysterectomy, whether it is abdominal, vaginal, laparoscopic, or robotic is still a major operation with recognized risks, which include potential damage to the adjacent organs (like bladder, bowel, and rectum), bleeding, infection, blood transfusion, blood clots to the legs and lungs, and a recovery period of 4-6 weeks. Just because a robotic hysterectomy was done, it doesn't mean it doesn't hurt, *and you still need to recover from having a major organ in your body removed*. The hospital time may be reduced with a laparoscopic approach to a hysterectomy (although not compared to a vaginal hysterectomy) but the body on a whole still needs time to recover.

Women deserve and demand a less invasive approach with a faster recovery and at less cost and less risk.

What is an ablation?

It is simply removing the lining of the uterus, whether it be with a radio frequency energy source (**Novasure**) or a thermal balloon technique (**Thermachoice**). A third choice, which is currently making a comeback with a retooled device, is the **Hydrothermal** (HTA) ablation. These are simple and effective techniques and have also been shown to reduce PMS (premenstrual syndrome and PMDD (premenstrual dysphoric disorder)as well.

Novasure and Thermachoice have emerged as the leading choices for treating the heavy bleeding and cramping after years of research and evolution of the technologies.We have passed by the older technologies of rollerball ablation and resection of the lining of the uterus, and laser of the inside of the uterus. Other technologies that have not quite made it to the fore front, because the data just isn't there, are cryoablation (freezing of the inside of the uterus), and microwaving the inside of the uterus.

The simplest and most effective treatments to date are the *Novasure* and *Thermachoice III* ablation procedures. The HTA is making a comeback with a redesigned cervical collar to prevent hot water leakage into the vagina during the procedure which was a problem with the old design.

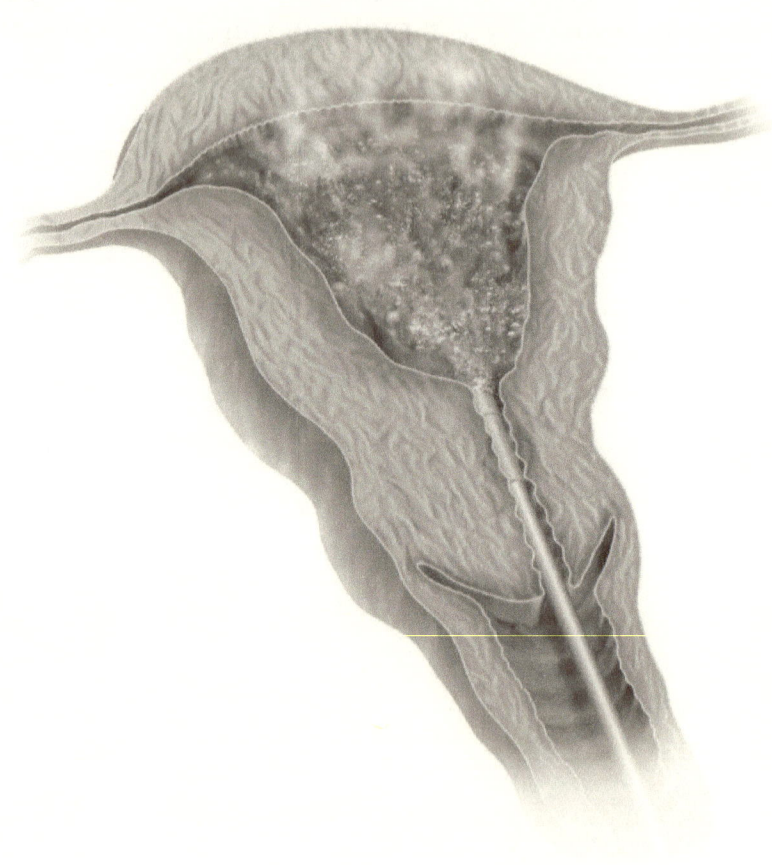

HTA (Hydrothermal) ablation.
Hot water freely circulating the uterus.

NOVASURE

What is Novasure?

Novasure is an endometrial ablation (EA) procedure that reduces heavy periods to light periods, or no periods at all. It is a **minimally-invasive office treatment alternative** to hysterectomy and a choice that avoids the potential side effects of hormone therapy. Ninety seconds of precisely controlled radio frequency energy is delivered through a thin handheld wand to remove (ablate) the lining of the uterus (endometrium) in the office setting using local or general anesthesia.

This unique procedure is quick and simple. It can be done with or without general anesthesia in the doctor's office. Once the procedure is over, most patients will have mild cramping and nothing much more. It is a minimally-invasive procedure that does not require incisions and can typically be done in less than 5 minutes for the Novasure. (10 minutes for the Thermachoice and HTA) Patients go home the same day and are back to work the following day. *Now, compare that to a hysterectomy!*

What is Thermachoice?

The Thermachoice III procedure does much the same things as Novasure but and takes a little longer with an eight minute completion time, and uses thermal heat as its energy source.

Why the excitement with these new technologies?

The facts speak for themselves.

Patients returning to normal levels of menstrual bleeding or low bleeding—78%
Amenorrhea (no period)—36%
Patients reporting satisfaction—92%
Patients reporting reduction in dysmenorrhea (cramping)—63%

While these numbers are the official 2006 statistics—our results, as well as others in private practice far exceed these, with PMS symptoms reduced over 65% of the time, amenorrhea (no period) in the range of 70-75%, and the cramping reduced to almost nothing in over 90%.

How does Novasure work?

The Novasure procedure can reduce or eliminate future menstrual bleeding by permanently removing the lining of the uterus through the quick delivery of radio frequency energy.

After slightly dilating your cervix (now done by hydrodilating the cervix with saline and eliminating the need for mechanically dilating the cervix with dilators, the inside of the uterus is visually inspected and measured, and then a slender fan-like device (Novasure)is gently inserted into the uterus.

This device gently expands and conforms to the dimension of your uterine cavity. Precisely measured radio frequency energy is delivered through the fan-like device for approximately 90 seconds.

The device is then retracted back into the wand and both are removed from your uterus. No part of the Novasure device remains inside your body after the procedure.

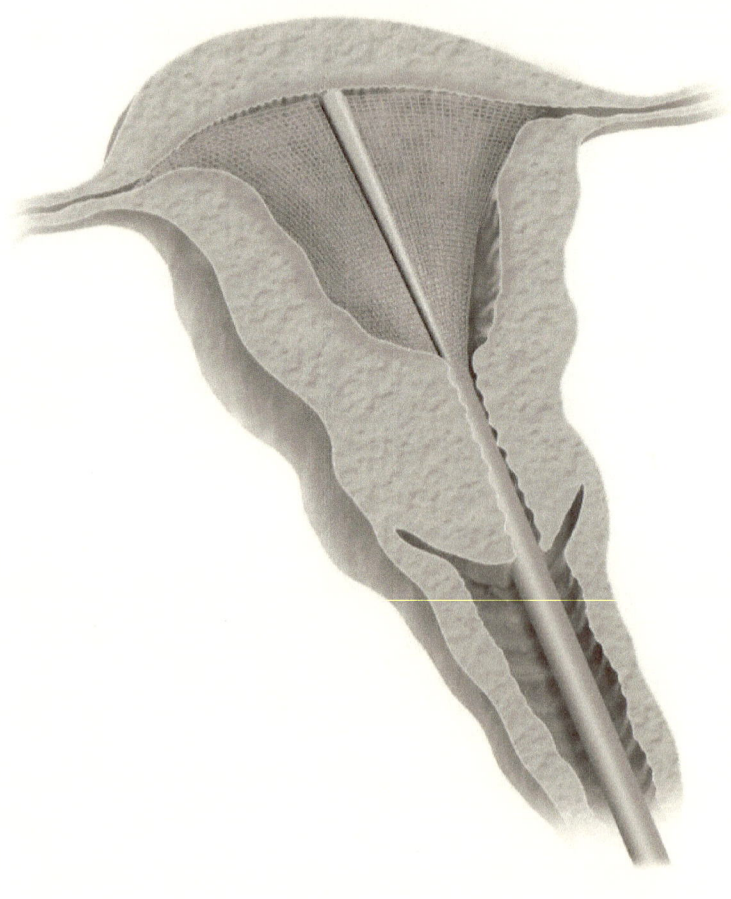

Novasure

Satisfaction rates are high.

Twelve months after Novasure, 93% of patients were satisfied with the results, and 97% said they would recommend Novasure to a friend.

Nearly 7 out of every 10 endometrial ablations (EA) performed are Novasure procedures and over one million had been performed by 2009, making Novasure the most popular EA technique at this time by the United States.

It is recommended as a treatment for heavy menstrual bleeding by the American College of OB/GYN (ACOG) and FDA approved.

Could the Novasure or Thermachoice procedure be right for me?

Women with menorrhagia (heavy periods) **who are finished having children** are candidates for an endometrial ablation. An endometrial biopsy (lining of the uterus sampled) to exclude abnormal tissue, and a sonohysterogram (filling the uterus with sterile water and doing a transvaginal ultrasound at the same time to check the shape of the cavity) must be done prior to the ablation.

The pap smear must also be up to date.

Can I still become pregnant after the Novasure or Thermachoice procedure?

There is still a small chance of becoming pregnant, and although it is only approximatley 1%, *it is necessary to use some form of birth control after your Novasure procedure.* Pregnancy may be dangerous for mother and child after an EA treatment. **The FDA has approved the ablation procedure for heavy bleeding, but not as a birth control indication.**

At this time, the Novasure procedure *is not indicated after the Essure procedure, only the Thermachoice III is. This may change in the near future as more data becomes available.*

After the Procedure

After EA with Novasure, you may feel some cramping and pain, this is normal. In most cases it may last for a few hours. You may have a watery and/or bloody discharge after the procedure and it could start anywhere from immediately after the procedure to a couple of weeks there after. The discharge might last only briefly or continue for up to a month. It is usually yellowish and thin. It could even come and go, and may increase after certain activities. This is quite normal and can be expected with any EA procedure.

Risks

Your doctor should explain the risks of the ablation in a pre-operative discussion. Some of the risks associated with EA procedures are a perforation in the uterus, bleeding, infection, or injury to organs within abdomen or around the uterus. These problems have been described in the literature but are very rare, even if you have had a C-section.

Tell your doctor if you have a cardiac pacemaker, defibrillator, or any other electrical device in your body.

THERMACHOICE III BALLOON SYSTEM

Thermal balloon therapy has evolved from the first device produced in 1997 and called Thermachoice I to Thermachoice II in 1999 to **Thermachoice III in 2006. Thermachoice III is the only FDA approved thermal balloon currently approved** for ablation.

Thermachoice ablation is also a good alternative to traditional hysterectomy or hormonal treatment for heavy menstrual bleeding and cramping, and differs from the Novasure (radio frequency cauterization technique) in that it provides a hot water treatment via a non latex balloon placed inside the uterus. The Thermachoice III System incorporates an impeller to help circulate fluid in the thermal balloon, distributing heat more efficiently.

While the Novasure and Thermachoice are similar in outcome results—there are some differences.

The energy source for the Novasure ablation is Bipolar Radio Frequency and the treatment cycle is approximately 90 seconds. The energy source for the Thermachoice is hot water (thermal heat), and the treatment cycle is 8 minutes plus a 2 minute "warm up."

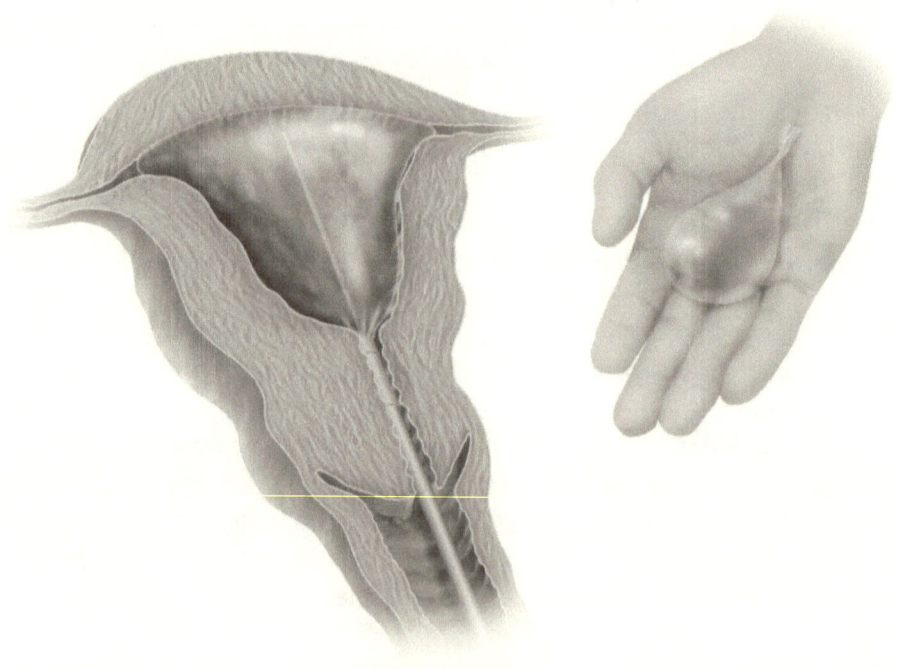

Theramachoice

Thermachoice III—here are some of the published data.

> Patients returning to normal levels of menstrual bleeding or lower—81%
> Patients experiencing amenorrhea (no period)—37%
> Patients reporting satisfaction—96%
> Patients experiencing reduction in cramping—89%

> (Data from Ethicon 2008)

The above numbers reflect part of the published data, and in our experience in our office, the rate of amenorrhea and reduced flow exceed the above.

Painful menstrual cramps go hand- in -hand in up to 93% of patients, so it is important to look at both of these symptoms when choosing an ablation technique.

At one year and three year follow-up, nearly 3 out of 4 women surveyed, who were treated with Thermachoice, reported reduction in menstrual cramping.

After 5 years:

> **Over 50% reported no pain associated with menses**
> **Over 30% reported only mild pain associated with menses**

To me, one of the main advantages of the Thermachoice balloon procedure is that it allows me to treat a uterine cavity that is irregular or distorted from fibroids or previous pelvic surgery.

It seems that there is a better outcome with the Thermachoice in patients with severe cramping, perhaps due to deeper tissue destruction from the transfer of thermal heat into the muscle of the uterus with Thermachoice.

A United States study published in the Journal of Gynecological Surgery by **Chape et al reported amenorrhea rates of 64% at 24 months and normal menstrual flow (with prior heavy flow) of 35% in 148 patients—very good indeed!**

A distinct advantage of the Thermachoice III System is the patient who has had an Essure (permanent birth control) procedure done and now elects to have an ablation performed. The manufacturer of the Novasure now lists the Novasure as a contradiction once the Essure has been performed, possible transfer of heat from the Novasure to the Essure microcoils and subsequent heat damage to the Fallopian tubes.

Outcomes after Thermachoice III

When comparing the Novasure and Thermachoice procedure, both show high levels of improvement in heavy bleeding and cramping. The amenorrhea rates are slightly higher in the Novasure group,(no head to head studies) but the reduction in cramping may be slightly better in the Thermachoice III group. In women with pre-existing premenstrual syndrome (PMS) more than half reported improvements in symptoms with both procedures. The Novasure is significantly quicker (90 Seconds) versus the 8 minutes for Thermachoice III, but no conclusive difference in pain or acceptability are noted in an excellent study by Clark et al. (Obstetrics and Gynecology Vol. 117, 2011.) Health related quality of life was improved after both treatments as were preexisting cramping and PMS symptoms in their study.

Local anesthesia vs. General anesthesia

Approximately one third of the 81 women in this same randomized controlled study by Clark would have preferred a general anesthesia in hind site, and that is why pre-operative counseling with the option of general anesthesia is so important.

All the women, (with the exception of just a couple in whom if failed totally for unknown reasons), who underwent ablation in our office have found it acceptable and would recommend it to a friend with a similar problem.

General anesthesia in the office is safely performed by a board certified anesthesiologist with IV medication, and there is no need for placing a tube down your throat. You will be monitored carefully and allowed to go home only when fully awake, alert, and comfortable.

In this same study by Clark et al 2011), he compared the Novasure to Thermachoice III. This is what he found:

> All the procedures were successfully completed in the Novasure group, where as two procedures (5%) were not completed in the Thermachoice III group due to discomfort.
>
> Complete destruction of the lining of the uterus was noted in 88% of the women with the Novasure (as visually noted by inspecting the uterus after the procedure, whereas complete destruction of the lining was noted in 58% of the women after Thermachoice III.
>
> There were no serious intraoperative complications in either group.
>
> The pain level during the procedure was much the same for both procedures. The pain level 1 hour after the procedure was less for the Novasure.
>
> There are no differences in the amount of time taken off from work.
>
> Amenorrhea rates were higher in the Novasure group, and reached statistical significance at 12 months.
>
> Both procedures showed high levels of improvement in heavy bleeding and cramping.In women with

preexisting premenstrual syndrome (PMS), more than half reported improvements in symptoms. **No women in either group reported using additional medical treatments to alleviate menstrual bleeding after surgery.**

CHAPTER THREE

LEAKY BLADDERS

Accidental loss of urine in women is common, but not talked about much until it reaches, well a leaking point . . . and sometimes, not even then! Bladder leaks are common in women as the muscle and tissue are often weakened by pregnancy, childbirth, trauma, radiation, surgery and hormone changes such as menopause. Urine leaks in women can occur simply by sneezing, coughing, laughing or lifting items.

The leak can be a small amount, enough to wear a liner at all times, or a spurt of urine with a cough, a sneeze, playing tennis, jumping on a trampoline, or just working out at the gym.

Actually, mild leakage affects most women at some time in their lives. Severe leakage is less common and affects at least one in ten women. Also, remember the U.S. population is aging and incontinence increases with age and 38-40% of women in the post menopausal years suffer from it.

In order to prevent urinary incontinence (leaking bladder), your bladder and urethra must be well supported by the pelvic muscle and issues.

How much leakage is important?

For an active woman virtually any accidental leakage is nasty! Whether it be leaking getting in and out of a car, during sex, at a social gathering, working in the garden or just rolling over at night—and it deserves attention. Some women have the false belief that loss of bladder control is a normal part of aging and think that nothing can be done to correct it, but often it can.

Women often do not tell their doctors about their symptoms of urine leakage if not asked. More than half of the women with symptoms do not seek medical help. Those women may not consider leakage to be a problem or they rely on absorbent pads to deal with the problem.

Normal urination occurs when a woman is able to empty her bladder when she feels the need to do so. In normal voiding, the bladder contracts and urine flows out the urethra. If she decides to stop the flow, she can if the sphincter or muscle valve that surrounds the neck of the bladder is intact. With an increase in bladder pressure, from for example, a cough or a jump, a leaky bladder will allow the urine to accidentally leak out. The sphincter or muscle surrounding the neck of the bladder cannot hold the urine in, because it is damaged.

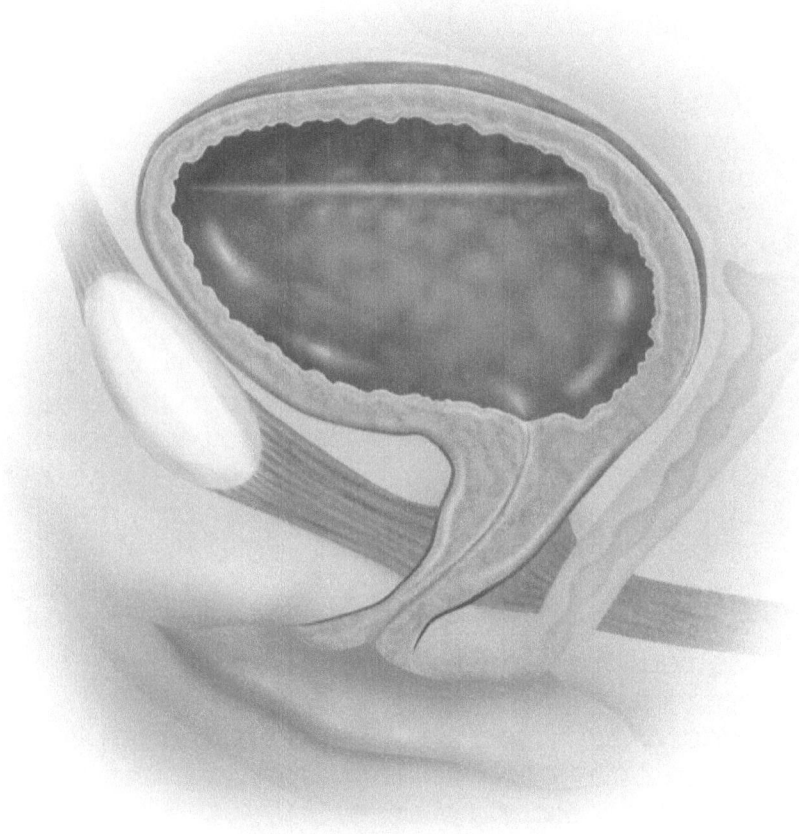

Normal continent bladder

Why does this happen?

The incontinent bladder has two main causes

1. Large babies
2. Genetic make up of the elastic and collagen fibers.

There are many causes of *urinary stress incontinence* as these conditions are collectively known.

1. Large babies
2. Genetic. The DNA that makes up the muscle fibers and collagen fibers are not programmed to be strong enough and the fibers do not hold up. Other causes such as radiation, radical surgery for cancer, hormone changes, may also cause urinary stress incontinence.
3. Prolapse (or falling out) of the uterus and bladder may cause incontinence as well. The supporting structures in the pelvis that hold the uterus and bladder in place are weakened from having large babies and/or the collagen and muscle fibers are genetically not strong, and this leads to accidental loss of urine.
4. Neuromuscular disorders, such as diabetes, stroke, multiple sclerosis, and polio.
5. Medications such as diuretics, drugs that contain caffeine.
6. Urinary Tract Infection. The bacteria in the bladder cause an irritation in the bladder wall and results in involuntary escape of urine.

What is urge incontinence?

The urgent need to urinate and the accidental loss of urine when the bladder is not full is called urge incontinence. The number one reason for this is *caffeine*. Caffeine is **the** major irritant of the bladder and you may have noticed that when you have a cup or two of coffee, or a can of coke, you may feel you have to go within 30 minutes or so. It is the caffeine that does this ! Remember, anything that has caffeine, like chocolate, cola drinks, tea, will cause bladder irritation. The carbonated drinks are a culprit as well.

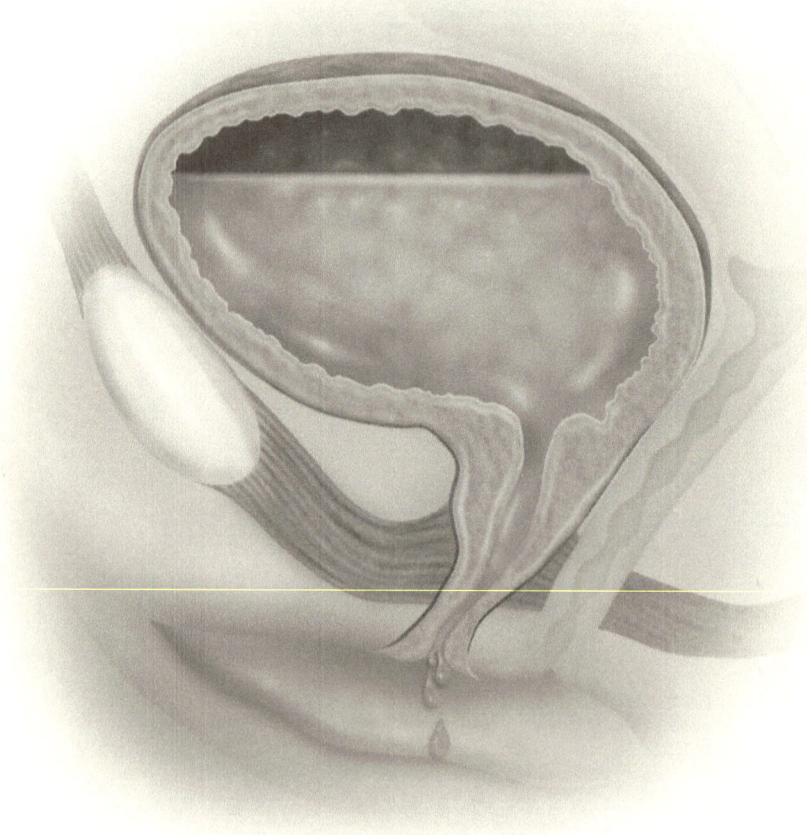

Incontinent bladder

How is the diagnosis of urinary stress incontinence made?

The most important part of the diagnosis is made by giving a good history and having a pelvic exam. As with most things in medicine, giving a good history helps get the right diagnosis! By explaining your symptoms in detail to the doctor, you are on your way to getting the correct diagnosis.

A diagnostic test can be done in the doctor's office, called a cystometrogram (CMG), and will confirm the diagnosis and rule out other causes of accidental urine loss.

A *cystoscopy* (looking inside the bladder through a thin lighted telescope) is not usually needed unless the diagnosis is difficult to come by, or the results of the CMG are not clear. The CMG will measure the volume of fluid the bladder can hold and at what pressure it will leak. Most importantly, it will tell the doctor if the diagnosis of urinary stress incontinence (USI) as suspected by the symptoms, history and physical exam is correct. **If the diagnosis of USI is confirmed it means a minimally invasive surgical procedure (a sling) will have an over 90% chance of success**.

Major advancements in the surgical treatment of USI have been made over the past few years and what used to be a major operation with an abdominal incision, 2-3 days in the hospital, and significant pain and expense, has now changed to a minimally invasive outpatient procedure that takes about fifteen minutes and requires a small incision in the vagina just below the bladder, the insertion of a polypropylene mesh as a "sling" to support the urethra, and 4-5 self absorbing stitches! The sucess rate is over 90%.

There has been a progression of techniqes to accomplish this "sling" or "hammock" to support the urethra, such as the "Monarc" "MiniArc" "Solex", and others. They all have an excellent track record (90% cure or major improvement), with little morbidity.

The most popular sling for years was the "TVT"(trans vaginal tape). It works well but has a higher rate of injury to the bladder and the blood vessels surrounding the bladder. The MonArc was then developed and appears just as good with less risks associated with it, but still the ocassional labial pain, inner thigh pain and gluteal pain. The current most popular slings are the MiniArc and Solex which are almost identical. They give cure rates over 90%, with minimal risk. *The MiniArc sling system* allows the physician to place an 8.5 cm long piece of polypropylene mesh under the urethra through a small incision (1.5 cm) in the vagina. This "sling" or "hammock" repositions and elevates the urethra in a position so that it mimics normal anatomy, to give more support and prevent accidental loss of urine.

There is minimal discomfort after the surgery and this minimally invasive procedure allows you to return to non-strenuous activities the day after surgery and no stitches need to be removed, the stitches are self absorbing. You should be able to return to your normal activities such as rigorous exercise, sexual intercourse, and heavy lifting in 4-6 weeks. The sling is designed to withstand the pressure of a cough that produces a tension of 5 lbs (normal cough exerts a tension of 2-3 pounds) and will not come out unless more than 8 lbs of tension is exerted on it. The mesh takes about 3 weeks to become a part of the body.

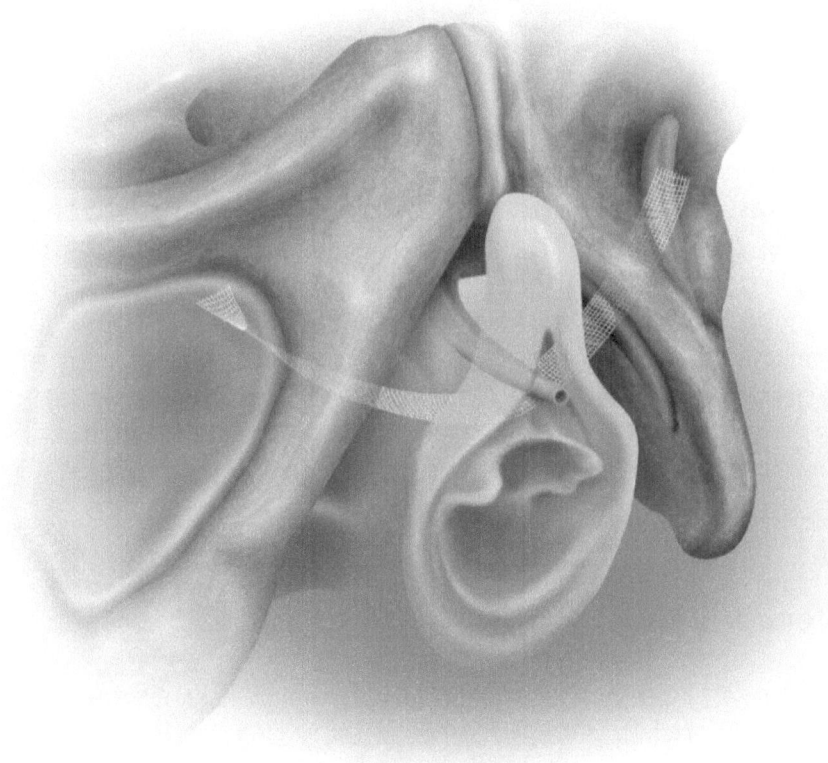

Vaginal sling supporting the urethra

When will I see results?

Most women will see results immediately following the procedure. It may take a day or so for the swelling to go down in some cases, but immediate improvement in the accidental loss of urine is the norm. You should be able to void immediately after surgery and will go home confident that you will not leak.

Important

Before you undergo this *mini sling* procedure, be sure you sit down with your doctor, look at pictures and diagrams of the anatomy, understand what the mesh looks and feels like, and know the potential risks associated with the operation. Be sure you know you may not get a 100% cure, because stress incontinence often has a mixed component, meaning, there may be additional factors at play, such as less than optimum tissue to work with, and there may be an urgency component that needs to be addressed with medication as well.

Potential Risks

As in any surgery, there are the potential risks of infection, bleeding, and damage to the nearby organs (such as the bladder and bowel). In the MiniArc there is also the risk that the mesh can erode through the vaginal wall and be exposed in the vagina (less than 2%). You will know if this happens by your partner complaining that "something" is scratching him during sex. The correction of this defect involves the use of an estrogen cream over the area for a month or two, and if that does not work a surgical revision of that area can be made.

FDA Warning

In 2011 the FDA warned that the mesh used in pelvic organ prolapse and incontinence procedures had a higher complication rate, especially with the potential to exposure in the vagina, and or, erosion into the bladder than was generally recognized. Although this potential risk is well known and not new, the FDA thought it necessary to reemphasize it in a so called "white paper". On close examination of their publication it refers mainly to the mesh repair of the prolapse of the top wall (anterior) of the vagina and the apex of the vagina with a larger mesh and not to the much smaller mesh used in the mini slings. There has been no modification to the indications or usage of the mini slings.

The MiniArc sling was introduced in 2007 and more than 75,000 procedures have been done. The MiniArc has become a favorite because it is simple, quick and has very good results and a low complication rate.

Between 2009 and 2010 there were 5 separate studies on the MiniArc that showed 85-94% success rate with the MiniArc in prospective studies.

CHAPTER FOUR

HORMONE THERAPY

At birth, there are about 500,000 to 1,000,000 potential eggs (follicles) in the ovaries, and this decreases steadily to approximately 1,000 at the age of menopause. As the number of follicles declines the cells that make the female hormones (estrogen and progesterone) decline as well and this leads to decreased production of Anti-Millerian Hormone (AMH) and Inhibin B and elevated Follicle Stimulating Hormone (FSH). Thus elevated FSH, and decreased AMH and Inhibin leads to the biochemical diagnosis of menopause.

So much for the chemistry! However, the most important way to diagnose menopause is by the symptoms of hot flashes, night sweats, dry vagina insomnia, irritability, dry eyes and skin changes. The diagnosis can be confirmed with the blood tests, as above.

What is the definition of menopause?

One year of no menses (periods) is the classic definition of menopause. The average age in American women is 51 years old. The transition to menopause, or the perimenopause, begins on average at 46 and ends on average at 51.

Some recent studies suggest that the genes you inherit from your mother are an important predictor as well. In the future, we will use the chemistry, genetics, historical, and environmental factors to predict more accurately when to expect that last period.

Approximately 1% of women will reach menopause by age 40, 10% by age 46, and 90% by age 55*

Premature ovarian failure, is now called Primary ovarian insufficiency and is defined as menopausal prior to age 40.

What are the actual menstrual cycle characteristics associated with the time to the final menstrual period? (FMP)

Early menopausal transition is defined by a change in menstrual cycle length by 7 or more days. This can last 7-8 years before the final menstrual period (FMP).

*The late menopausal transition** is defined by two or more skipped periods or no period at all for 60 days or more. This begins approximately 3-4 years prior to the FMP. About 10% of women will have regular periods up to their FMP.

* Menopause Medicine, May 2011

The hot flash

Hot flashes are the most common symptom related to the menopause transistion. The frequency, severity, and duration vary in different populations. In Europe and North America, hot flashes affect around 70% of women and persist for an average of 2 to 5 years, although some 20% of women continue to flash into their 70's and 80's.

What causes the hot flash* ?

We really are not sure! It seems to be a complex process of not just estrogen decline, which is the initial step, but decline

of serotonin, noradrenalin, dopamine, acetylcholine, GABA, and others.

*Editorial: Menopause, Vol 16. No. 5, 2009

Hormone Therapy

This chapter on hormone therapy for menopausal women is not intended to be a comprehensive treatise or the final word to resolve all the disagreements on hormone therapy ! In the next few pages, I would like to tell you in a "nutshell" what you should know in order to make an informed decision on whether to use hormones in your menopause.

The First Hormone Experiment 1898

Back in 1898, German doctors fed fresh cow ovaries to a young woman experiencing severe hot flashes after her ovaries had been removed—and she felt better, the severe hot flashes got better! This was a milestone in the use of "hormones" to treat menopausal symptoms leading to commercially prepared drugs that we have today.

By the 1960's, pharmaceutical companies were making products that were acceptable to women and women were all in favor of "staying young forever" with these new drugs.

The next major event in the research of hormone therapy for women began in 1991 when the National Institute of Health embarked on the Women's Health Initiative (WHI). This was a $625 million study that involved 40 well recognized medical centers across the United States that would examine the risks and benefits of menopause hormones, calcium and vitamin D supplements, and low fat diets. 26, 000 women were recruited for the hormone research part which I will confine this section to. **Of special significance is that the government funded the study not big pharmaceutical companies!**

The study was stopped, quite dramatically with press releases and media blitzes, in 2002, because it showed that the hormone drug used in the study, *PremPro* (Premarin plus Provera) increased the risk of breast cancer, heart attacks, and strokes.

The media went crazy with this information that they did not know how to interpret, and played it out of context totally because it was—*NEWS*. They have as much admitted so, but the blame lies also with doctors who allowed it to happen and did not make sure that the information was reported in a responsible way.

In the table below you will see what the data says. This is the data you need to understand as to what the risk of taking hormone therapy is, and what the benefits are.

Landmarks from Two Decades of Study

1991 National Institues of Health embarks on a study of menopause hormones after observational data suggest that women who use hormones have lower rates of heart disease.

2002 Part of the Women's Health Initiave is stopped after women in the study taking estrogen plus progestin (E+P) show higher rates of heart attack, stroke, and breast cancer. Millions of women abandoned hormones overnight.

2003 Women taking E+P are not protected from mild memory loss; they are found to be at increased risk for developing dementia.

2004 The second W.H.I. hormone study is stopped one year early because women taking estrogen only show a small increased risk of stroke.

2006 An updated analysis of the estrogen-only trial in women who have had a hysterectomy shows hormone therapy does not increase the risk of breast cancer.

2007 Combined data from both hormone trials suggest that timing of therapy may affect risk; hormones may reduce heart disease in women who start therapy closer to menopause.

2009 Women using E+P for more than about five years double their annual risk of breast cancer. It appears to be 26% higher than women who did not take hormones, but it is still only 0.008, which is not even statistically significant but the risk is higher than previously thought.

2011 Follow-up of women in the estrogen-only study shows those who took just estrogen had 23 percent fewer breast cancers; younger estrogen users had 46 percent fewer heart attacks. This sounds crazy, but is published in peer review journals.

The Highlights

The initial WHI data has been dissected over and over since 2002 and new information keeps on coming out. I will try to keep it simple.

In April 2011, the American Medical Association reported *that certain women who used Premarin (estrogen) only, (not the Provera) during the study had markedly reduced risk for breast cancer and heart attacks.* This is great news. Why? Because it is telling us it is unlikely that the estrogen alone causes breast cancer. It may be the combination of estrogen plus progesterone (E+P) or it may be the Provera that is the catalyst.

This subset of data from the WHI published in 2011 showed that in the estrogen-only study; these women who took estrogen alone had 23% fewer breast cancers and younger women had 46% fewer heart attacks.

The current thinking is that estrogen does not cause a new breast cancer to form. If a breast cancer is already there—and remember it takes approximately 10 years for a breast cancer to become palpable, and the breast cancer is estrogen sensitive (receptor positive) it will make the breast cancer grow larger and quicker—but there is no conclusive data to say it makes a new breast cancer form.

New data also suggests that the ideal time to take hormone therapy is the first 10 years of menopause. It is at this time that the coronary arteries will benefit the most. If hormone therapy is started in the 60's, it may well be harmful to the heart and also may increase the risk of stroke in these women, but starting hormone therapy between 50-59 years does not increase heart disease risk and probably decreases it. *

It is important to understand that all women are different, not just medically or metabolically, but psychologically and physiologically. "One size does not fit all" in hormone therapy. Individualization is the key and each woman needs to understand what *her individual* risk is, and what *her* options are, and then decide if she wants to use the hormones.

Let me emphasize, use of these hormones is elective. We are talking about a quality of life issue here. We are not talking about saving a life or prolonging a life—we are attempting to improve the way you feel, reduce the hot flashes and night sweats so you sleep better, reduce the discomfort and pain of intercourse, make you feel more sensuous, improve libido, improve self image, and as so many patients have told me "get my life back"

Life is all about risk taking. Whether we consciously acknowledge it or not whatever we do involves some kind of risk.

Taking hormone therapy also involves some risk. What is important is, does the benefit of taking hormones outweigh the risk *in your* particular case.

As a comparison, we have to drive the car to buy food, get the kids to school, go to work, so the benefit is obvious. We also use the car electively all the time to go places not only because of necessity, but because we want to. *We elect to.*

And so it is with hormone therapy. There are some women who do not feel the need to use hormones—their quality of life as defined above is just fine, so the risk of taking hormones may not be justified for them. On the other hand, there are women who are quite miserable from the lack of estrogen and a small increase in the risk of breast cancer is a small price to pay for "getting their life back."

It is important for us not to judge those who want to use hormone therapy. I have often heard the statement "My husband doesn't want me to take hormones." Or, "I have just read this book or magazine that says you should never take hormones!" Please do your homework, use this book to know what questions to ask, and then decide for yourself ! My point, you must understand what the data says.

Here again is my oversimplified explanation. According to the best data we have and that is the WHI data, the risk of breast cancer is increased 26% in women who take Estrogen and Progesterone (E & P) compared to those that do not. (10,000 women in hormone group and 10,000 in placebo group over 5 years.) There are 8/10,000 more women (0.008) who will get breast cancer taking E & P over 5 years, compared to those that do not. After a follow up of 11 years in those that took estrogen and progesterone, there was an

increase finding of breast cancer of 0.42% compared to the placebo group 0.34% The frequency of mammography was the same in both groups.

Same for heart attacks and strokes.

Blood clots are increased by 16/10,000 compared to those that did not.

24% of women with breast cancers had positive lymph nodes in the E + P group, compared to 16% in the placebo group.

Breast cancer mortality was increased in women taking estrogen and progesterone compared with women taking placebo. The absolute risk was 2.6 deaths in the estrogen and progesterone group, and 1.3 in the placebo group.

What about the Estrogen patch and the gels? (Transdermal or vaginal rings).

This is without a doubt the way to go. The estrogen used in the transdermal patch and gels is a Natural, Bio-Identical Estrogen. This means it is exactly the same estradiol that your ovaries made when they were in full production.

The main advantage of this transdermal estrogen or vaginal estrogen ring is that it is neutral on the clotting system and may not increase the risk of blood clots and strokes. Also important is that this mode of application delivers an even steady blood level through the day so that the highs and lows (which can be felt in the form of hot flashes are night sweats and fatigue) are minimized.

In contrast to the transdermal products, when taking a tablet by mouth such as Premarin, the tablet needs to be absorbed first in the digestive tract, then it goes through the liver where the blood clotting proteins are stimulated to increase the clotting factors that are responsible for clots and strokes.

A less talked about fact is that concentration of estrogen from the tablet, will peak in 2 hours after ingestion by mouth and then rapidly drops off—so that the dosage of the pill tends to be higher than necessary to prevent the hot flashes reappearing in a few hours.

There is a mantra, which is more of a legal one than a medical one, that says the **"lowest dose for the shortest period of time"** is certainly one to respect, but it is more of a legal opinion than a medical one. It may not be harmful to leave someone on hormones for an extended period of time with close surveillance, if she does not do well off them and her quality of life is seriously affected off the hormone therapy.

The vaginal application of estrogen, such as the vaginal rings (FemRing, Estring) is equally effective and as safe as the transdermal patches and gels.

It is important to know that one type of estrogen, whether it be *Estrone, Estradiol, or Estriol* is not safer than another when it comes to breast cancer. There is no data to conclusively show that any one of these three natural estrogen's is better for you, *except it is appreciated that transdermal or vaginal application is associated with less strokes and blood clots. There is more and more data to support this approach. Estriol is the weakest of the 3 estrogens and by far the most expensive.*

Progesterone

The most natural form of progesterone is **micronized progesterone** that comes in a capsule called **Prometriu**m. It is an excellent product and is most effective when used in oral or vaginal form. Some women find it messy when used in the vagina, so it is used most often by mouth. **The micronized progesterone protects the uterus from cancer and must be used if estrogen's are prescribed. If estrogen are used alone there is a very real risk of uterine cancer over time.**

Of added benefit is that some of the progesterone gets converted to estrogen as well, so it can fine tune the estrogen therapy as well.

Vaginal Estrogen Therapy

It is effective and well tolerated for the treatment of vulva-vaginal atrophy.

Estradiol tablets, creams, and rings are available. There is limited absorption of estrogen into the blood stream or into the uterus from the vaginal preparations.

Side Effects of ET/EPT

If the right hormone preparation and the right dosage is used, there is seldom a side effect. Fine tuning the dose is sometimes necessary, but you as the patient should be bringing this to the attention of your gynecologist within the first two weeks of therapy.

Uterine bleeding is not what we see very often anymore. If it occurs, changing the dosage or the preparation will stop it.
Breast tenderness (sometimes enlargement). This is from the estrogen and usually goes away within a month. If not, the estrogen needs to be reduced.
Nausea is very uncommon.
Abdominal bloating. Seen more often with Premarin than the transdermals.

Fluid retention in extremities—just a slight amount of swelling usually in the lower legs and feet is sometimes seen, again not common.

Headaches If you are sure it is from the hormones, tell the doctor and try something different usually with a lower estrogen dosage.

Dizziness and *mood changes* are seldom due to the hormones, but if there is no other reason for these symptoms look to the doctor for a different preparation.

Who should not take hormone therapy?

Undiagnosed or abnormal vaginal bleeding

Personal history of breast cancer (with some exceptions, like painful intercourse, and then a vaginal preperation would be appropriate.)Active blood clots in the legs, lungs, or blood vessels of the heart. If there is a history of clots—this needs to be discussed. Liver disease, hepatitis, pregnancy are also contraindications to hormone therapy.

The information above is from the WHI study that studied *Premarin and Provera* and not the transdermal or vaginal estrogen, and not the natural progesterone, Prometrium. The reason I mention this, is that there are women who are quite miserable with hot flashes, night sweats, and painful intercourse who will choose to use a very low dose transdermal or vaginal estradiol product (with or without the natural progesterone) in spite of a personal history of breast cancer or blood clots. This is where the *individualization* comes in, and working with a knowledgeable doctor to find relief is so important.

One of the newest advances is the use of vaginal DHEA cream or suppositories to counter the effects of the dry vagina and low libido. (painful intercourse.) The product has very good support in the scientific literature and works by being converted into estrogen and testosterone in the vagina, and it remains local in the vagina, so it hardly, if at all, will raise the blood levels of estrogen or testosterone. I will have a compounding pharmacist make it and dispense it, and so far the results are very good. We have many repeat patients saying it not only helps restore the vagina, but it increases libido as well.

A frequent question that comes up is "how do I know how much estrogen and progesterone to take?" Is there a test to help? Is the saliva test helpful?

The answer is quite simply, *you are the test!!*

We do not need to do blood tests or saliva tests to know if you are doing well ! If your symptoms are gone and you feel better—we are there! Only in a very few exceptional cases do we need to do the blood tests. We occasional encounter someone who is difficult to get symptom/side effect free, and then there are women who cannot seem to get enough estrogen, we call these women *Estro-holics*. It seems their metabolism of estrogen is just different and it is difficult to know how much estrogen they need. This being the case, we will measure the estrogen in the blood and make adjustments.

In spite of the promotion of the salivary tests for the hormones, there is very little scientific support for them. For example, if the estrogen level in the saliva is known—what does it tell us about the estrogen in the rest of the body?

Estrogen, along with progesterone, cortisol, testosterone and other hormones is secreted in pulses, resulting in fluctuating blood levels. Research* was conducted to determine whether the flucuations noted in salivary assays are the same as in blood assays. **The results show there was a fairly good correlation for within-subject analysis, but a poor correlation between subjects**. As such, there is no standard concentration of hormone levels in saliva that can be used to set values. So what does this mean? **It means that salivary hormone levels do not necessarily reflect concentrations in the blood. This brings me back to you—the test model. You are the test—how you feel on the hormones is what counts—not the hormone levels in the saliva or blood.**

Bioidentical Hormones

The term "bioidentical hormones" means different things to different people. To scientists and health care providers, bioidentical hormones are those that are chemically identical to the hormones produced by your ovaries during the reproductive years. There are three estrogens that are produced by the ovaries :Estrone (E1), Estradiol (E2), Estriol (E3) as well as testosterone and progesterone.

Please remember these custom compounded hormones are not FDA approved and they are not safer than the FDA regulated hormones. They are not more physiological or safer simply because they are made in the private laboratory of a pharmacy. My own approach to the custom-compounded hormones is not to be critical of an "alternative" approach or a "novel" approach to individualize a therapeutic product for a patient, but we do need a reality check to make sure the information the patient gets is accurate and the product is safe, the quality top notch, and it is what it is supposed to be.

What is the effect of estrogen on the skin, hair, ears, eyes, and joints?

These questions come up all the time—especially with regard to aging, so here is a short review.

Skin

Hormones play an important role in the physiology of the skin. Acne is due to the increase in the ratio of androgen to estrogen and this leads to an increase in the sebum production and acne. Adult women with acne almost always had acne as a teenager. An increase in the androgen to estrogen means that there is relatively more androgen present in the menopause—therefore the acne.

There is a significant decline in skin collagen and skin thickness as the estrogen (age increase) declines. About 30% of the skin collagen is lost during the first five years after menopause and it continues over the next 20 years at a slower rate. There is also an increase in skin elasticity, wrinkling, laxity as the menopause progresses.

Hair

Some women experience thinning of the hair on the scalp or unwanted hair on the face in midlife. The reason for this is mostly unknown.

Hirutism

5-15% of women will develop coarse facial hair and this is due to the overproduction of androgen by the ovary, such as in polycystic ovarian syndrome. We must exclude the intake of androgens (perhaps used to stimulate libido) and some unusual enzymatic aberration like 5 alpha-reductase hyperactivity (laboratory test).

Another concern is the appearance of fine hairs ("Peach Fuzz") on the face. This growth of unwanted hair is common and sometimes starts long before menopause, so is likely genetic in origin.

Eyes

Dry eye syndrome is a common complaint of postmenopausal women. Blurred vision, increased tearing, swollen and reddened eyelids are common too. Unfortunately there is no quick fix here with hormone therapy, although some women have reported improvement on HRT especially when methyltestosterone is used. At this time, HRT is not recommended to treat dry eye syndrome as such.

Hearing changes

There is some evidence that estrogen would appear to have a positive effect on hearing in the postmenopausal women.

Arthritis and Joint Pain

There are over 100 causes of arthritis in women after the menopause. And there is no clear data that says hormone therapy works here. Anectdotally, I have seen patients who say their joint pain improved on HRT, more so in the Asian population.

Memory

The controversy here, is if HT increases or decreases the risk of dementia the data originates from early observational studies before the WHI study. These observational studies suggested that HT reduced the risk of dementia. In contrast, the WHI study (women were on average of 63 years old) found that *the initiation of HT later in life increased* the risk of dementia. This has led to the theory that using HT in the perimenopause or early menopause may lower the risk of dementia, but starting HT over the age of 63 years may indeed worsen it. *Age matters!!!*

Bones

There is clear evidence that estrogen therapy prevents osteoporotic fractures. [OBG Management May 2011. Vol 23 #5]

I have tried in this chapter on Hormone Therapy to present the data from the WHI and it's update, in a digestable form, so that you can use the information to make an informed decision on whether to use hormone therapy for your menopausal symptoms—or not. It is not a simple matter, so please do not be discouraged by the enormity and complexity of the studies.

I will emphasize again that the key in your decision to use hormone therapy is to individualize your therapy and work with your gynecologist to find the right approach for you. Every year come in for an update and check up, and stay up to date on your mammograms, and self breast exams if you can.